Made in the USA
Middletown, DE
09 October 2022

12397213R00057